Diabetes

How it can control your life

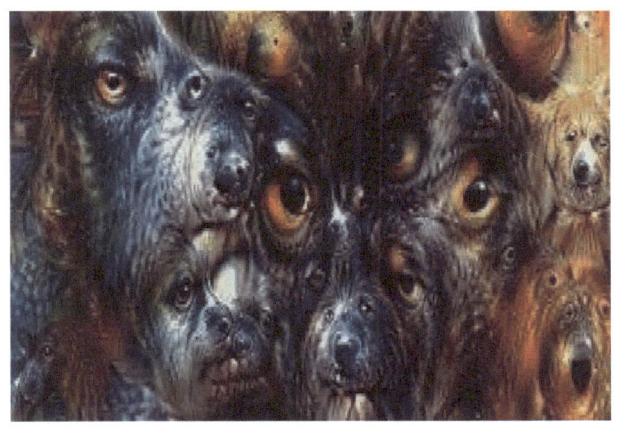

Diabetes comes with many faces

Diabetes how it can control your life

Dedication

This book is dedicated to my mom "Sandra F. Luckett" and to all diabetics. May God be with you all through this terrible battle with this silent killer.

Tammy Thomas

Other books by the Author

Simple Poetry Expressions

Drugs Crack Cocaine and How it Can Ruin Your Life

Isaiah Let's Try Something New

I am A Diva and I Rock

From a boy to a Man to a Leader

Hermanology

The Same Thang That Makes You Laugh Will Make You Cry

Diabetes

Words with a Vision" coming soon"

My Life My Surroundings and My Opinion"coming soon"

Diabetes how it can control your life

Contact Information

Facebook:https://www.facebook.com/tam.thomas.90?fref=ts

Twitter: https://twitter.com/Taymoes1

Instagram: Taymoes1

Amazon-www.amazon.com

website:t-thomas.wix.com/t-thomas

Tammy Thomas

Acknowledgement

I want to thank you James Scott because you are a very hard worker I told you what my dreams were and what I wanted to accomplish, you told me that I can do it and that I am well on my way. Even though he was going through some tough times this man stayed on his job of helping me accomplish my dreams so that I can rock like the Diva that I am, Thank you so much. If anyone is looking for some help publishing their books get in Touch with him at jamesscott799@yahoo.com he will get the job done!

Diabetes how it can control your life

God has the situation undercontrol

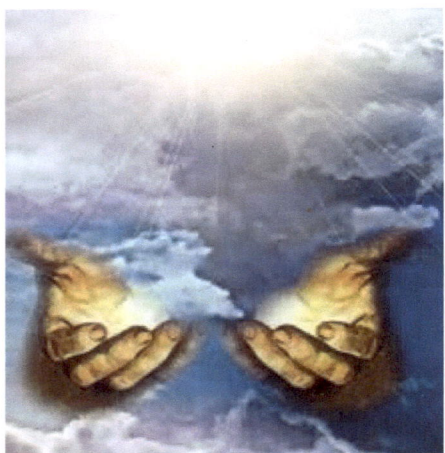

To all fighting this disease this is just some information provided to you requested by my mother, because she doesn't understand why this is happening to her, but she feels that you can save yourself.

Tammy Thomas

My Mom

This is one courageous strong black woman I don't know if I could ever whether the storm the way she whether hers. My Mom Sandra Fay Luckett known as the lady that loves to feed the neighborhood. **She Is a Diva and I rock!**

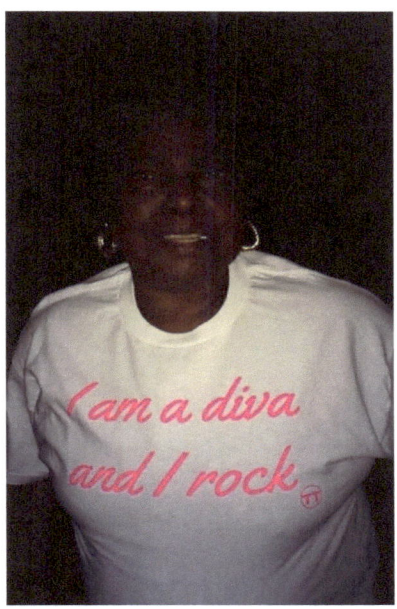

Diabetes how it can control your life

Type1 diabetes, once known as juvenile diabetes or insulin-dependent diabetes, is a chronic condition in which the pancreas produces little or no insulin, a hormone needed to allow sugar (glucose) to enter cells to produce energy. The far more common type2 diabetes occurs when the body becomes resistant to insulin or doesn't make enough insulin.

Various factors may contribute to type1 diabetes, including genetics and exposure to certain viruses. Although type 1 diabetes usually appears during childhood or adolescence, it also can begin in adults.

Despite active research, type 1 diabetes has no cure. But it can be managed. With proper treatment, people with type 1 diabetes can expect to live longer, healthier lives than did people with type1 diabetes in the past.

Tammy Thomas

Type 2 diabetes, Very Important:
A. the pancreas stops making the proper amount of insulin.

B. the body doesn't have the proper and/or the liver produces too much sugar.

Treating type 2 diabetes make sure you keep your blood sugar level at whatever you and your health care provider comes up with you don't want your blood sugar to be low. Lowering and controlling blood sugar may help prevent or delay complications. Such as:

- heart problems
- kidney problems
- blindness
- amputation

Diabetes how it can control your life
Dealing with Diabetes

Diabetes management requires a lot of time and effort, especially in the beginning.

You need to have your family and your friends to pull together for support.

Alone with everything else that I am going through I can and will say that I am a true survivor and I will fight this until the very end.

I know that God has me and he will not let me walk the through the greens pastures by myself.

Tammy Thomas

Diabetes can affect your emotions both directly and indirectly. Poorly controlled blood sugar can directly affect your emotions by causing behavior changes, such as irritability. Diabetes may also make you feel different from other people. And there may be times you feel resentful that you always have to incorporate diabetes planning in everything you do. This can also be very depressing, stressful on you and your family. You must stay on top of it like clockwork because one minute it can be too high and the next minute it can be too low.

Diabetes how it can control your life

Staying on top

Keep up with your health from Head to Toe. Dealing with Diabetes can become a Lifetime/threatening complications. All body parts can be affected by diabetes.

1. **Make yourself, your first priority and commitment to managing your diabetes**
2. **Keep the same routine when it comes down to administer your meds at the same time every day.**
3. **Every day you should check your feet and keep them oiled.**
4. **Make sure you keep your blood pressure**
5. **Take stress seriously**
6. **Exercise**
7. **Good diet**

Tammy Thomas

The cause it diabetes

The exact cause of type 1 diabetes is unknown. In most people with type 1 diabetes, the body's own immune system — which normally fights harmful bacteria and viruses — mistakenly destroys the insulin-producing (islet) cells in the pancreas. Genetics may play a role in this process, and exposure to certain environmental factors, such as viruses, may trigger the disease.

Diabetes how it can control your life

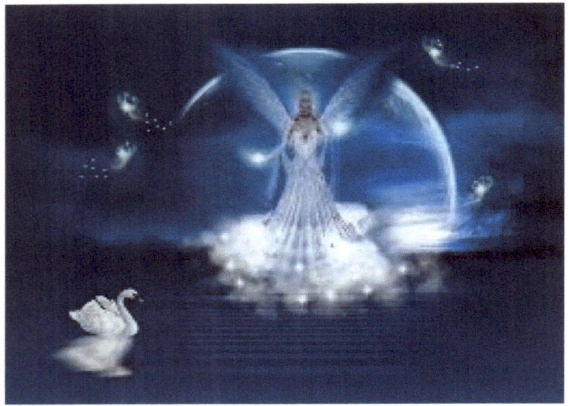

Sandra F. Luckett is protected by God Angels; they are watching over her. Thank you Jesus.

Tammy Thomas

About my mom Sandra Luckett

She 'Sandra Luckett' has been dealing with other disease that comes along with diabetes for years and every year it seems as if something else comes about. I have been eating what I want and not taking this disease seriously because it was hard for me to accept the fact that I was a diabetic and all these other problem were coming along with it. mom also have kidney problems which mom currently on dialysis three times a week, Chronic Vascular Disease which is stopping mom blood flow from getting to the necessary areas in my body to function properly, High blood pressure which they are having a hard time controlling mom's highs and

lows. Digestion problems that mom was recently hospitalized and was throwing up bile which

Diabetes how it can control your life

mom has a calcium build up at the top part of her stomach that doesn't allow the blood to throw through correctly which upset the small intestines alone with the high blood pressure that makes her intestine sick and they don't pass the bile through correctly so it end up comes up through the mouth as a result to help her they end up putting the Gtube down her nose several time to pump the toxic out of her stomach. The Kidney disease which has something to do with my aggressive Vasculitis, an inflammation of blood vessels that has so much build up in them that blood can't pass through properly. I still produce some urine. I attend dialysis three days a week. I have to test my blood sugar four times a day and blood pressure twice a day. If my mom or any diabetic blood sugar is over 180 it causes your wounds to heal slowly. I have had a numerous amount of high blood

Tammy Thomas

pressure along with my blood sugar being out of control to lead to many other problems such as causing the wounds to heal which I stepped on a nail and she soaked it in peroxide and it spread so fast that it took the attention off the finger which was rotting off due to a scratch from her dog "Romeo" and my big toe on my right foot which I stumped. My foot that I stepped on the nail ended up leading to an amputation up to a little under the knee; it is healing slowly due to the power levels of my blood sugar. But my mother is a strong black woman that is not going down without a fight, there was a couple times we thought we were going to lose her and she pulls through every time. I share this with you because if you are a diabetic I want you to take care of yourself so that you or your family don't have to go through what we have to endure during this situation and lord

Diabetes how it can control your life

knows my mom deserves a medal even the doctors said that she is one tough cookie "smile" So we ask you to please know yourself, your body, your mind, your soul and most of important know your worth. Treat yourself like a diamond. Don't let the diabetes take over your body and your life you can live with it but if you don't take care of yourself it can kill you fast or slow your choice. Stay stress free and surround yourself around positive people.

Tammy Thomas
The Kidney

Kidney disease/ failure also called renal failure occurs when your kidneys suddenly become unable to filter waste products from your blood, kidneys lose their filtering ability, dangerous levels of wastes may build up in your body which may cause, your blood's chemical makeup may get out of balance. This disease can be fatal and develop in a couple minutes, hours, and/days and requires intensive treatment. You may or may not continue to produce urine. Then you end up doing at least three days a week on dialysis. The cause of kidney failure comes from improper blood flow to the kidney." See references for more details"

Diabetes how it can control your life

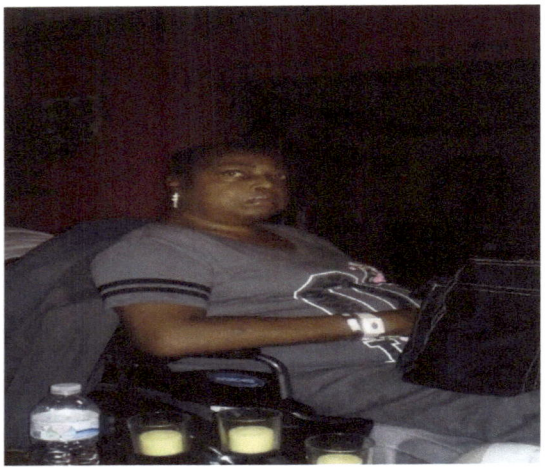

I am very serious. I/we didn't believe, but I/we am a believer now. Don't too late, get checked out, keep your body examined, watch your every step and the most important thing is to always keep shoes on your feet.

A wake Call

Tammy Thomas

The photos that we have present some may not be able to stomach them but this is reality and we deal with this on a daily basis.

Photos of what diabetes causes reality check. Please take this disease seriously it's no joke

Diabetes how it can control your life

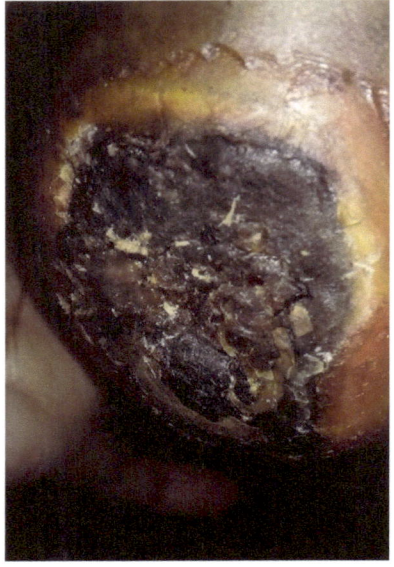

Because of stepping on a nail.

Tammy Thomas

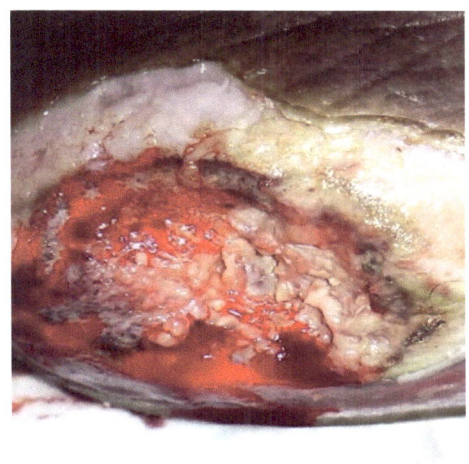

After cleaning and removing dead skin to try and save it before the amputation.

Diabetes how it can control your life

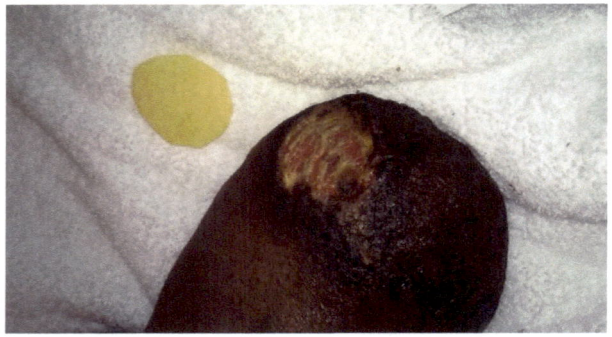

The stump is finally healing after about 4 months

Tammy Thomas

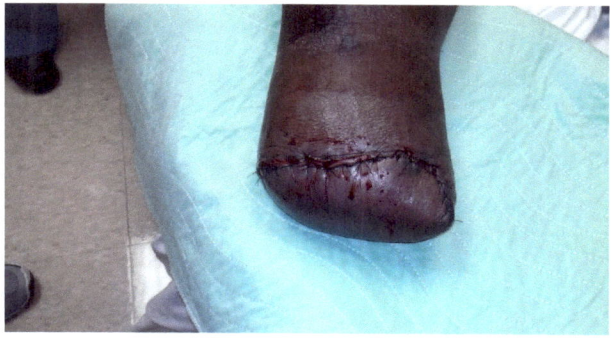

The nail lead to this. My mom lost her leg

This started from a dog scratch

Diabetes how it can control your life

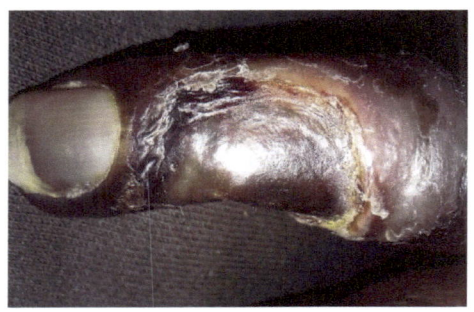

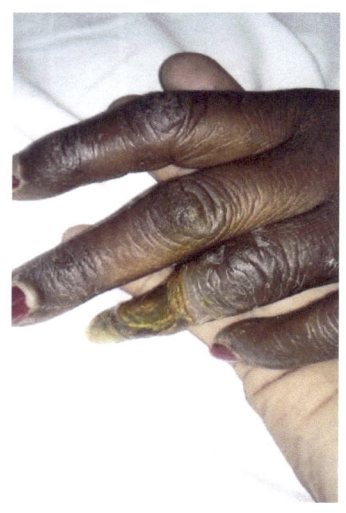

Tammy Thomas

They called it dry gangrene and this would eventually rot off.

This finger started off with a scratch from a dog. It is what you call dry gain green and the finger will just have to rot off do to my vascular disease and diabetes. They can't do anything for it because of the poor circulation problem that would cause it not to heal or take a long time to heal. This what a wound look like that's not healing properly because on uncontrolled Blood sugar levels

Diabetes how it can control your life

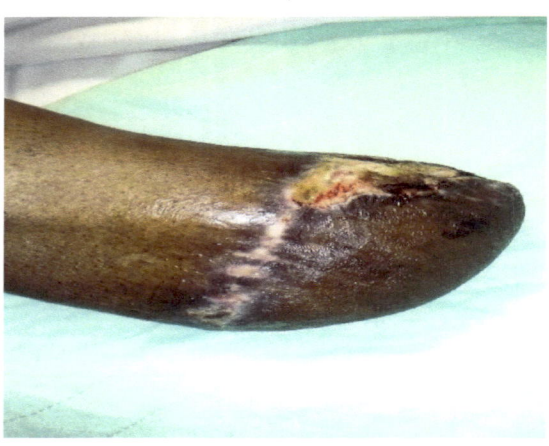

The stump healing is being prolonged due to poor blood sugar management. "The blood sugar is not controlled"

Tammy Thomas

Front side of

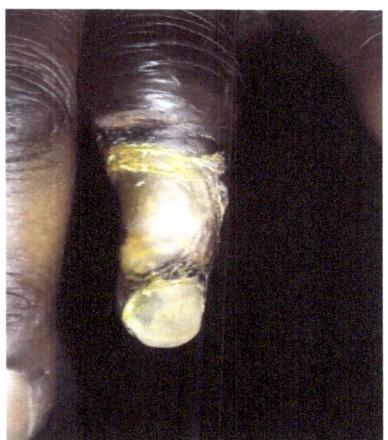

A wake up call!! Look at the finger this has been going on over 6mths dry gain green and now another finger with drainage Hummmmm!

Diabetes how it can control your life

There are a lot of people that don't care for the pictures but there are some that appreciates them. It gives them an idea of what could happen if you do not take care of the smallest cut when it comes down to diabetes.

The stump steady drains the unhealed wound. It's very important to stay on top of the dressing changes as directed by the Doctor in charge of care.

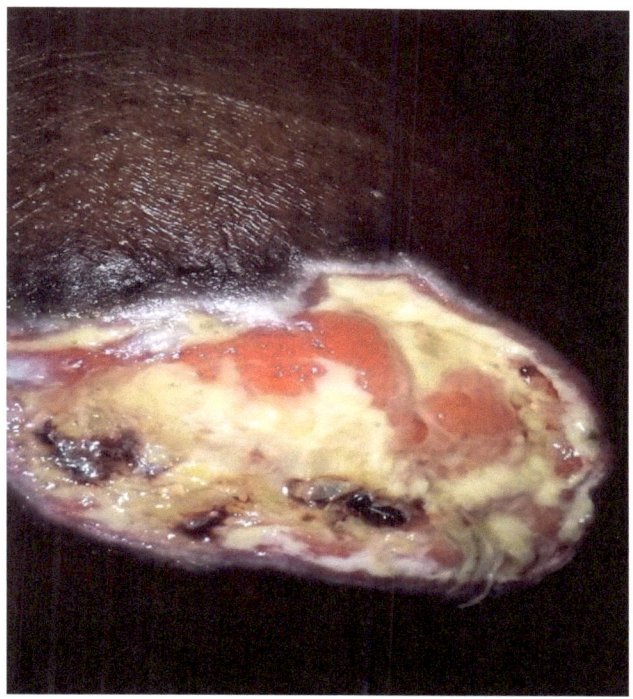

Poor healing due to blood sugars and lack of blood flow.

Diabetes how it can control your life

Drainage from the stump/wound still healing from surgery December 2015 The changes have went from 24 hours to every 8 hours. They changed the dressing changes at least 4 times and there will be many more.

Tammy Thomas

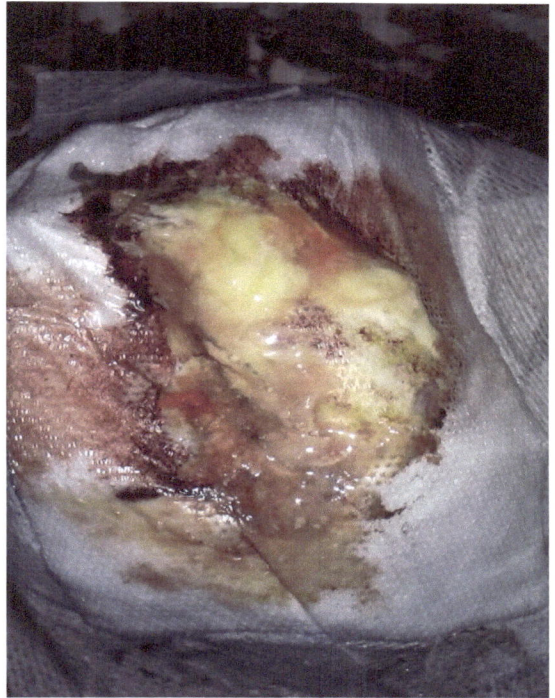

Drainage we deal with on a daily basis.

Dressing changes and mediation must be taken and/or changed as direction by the Doctor.

Diabetes how it can control your life

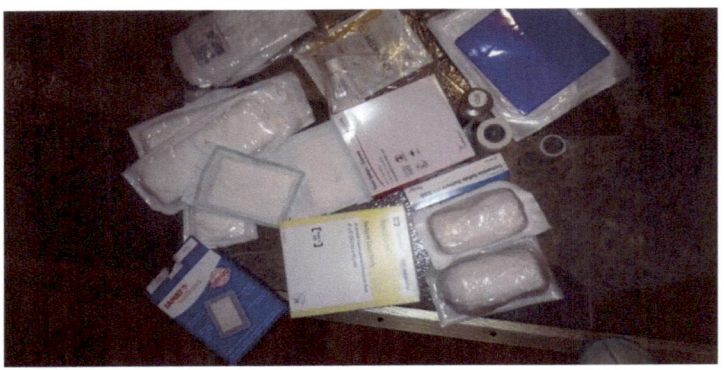

Dressing changes A lot

Tammy Thomas

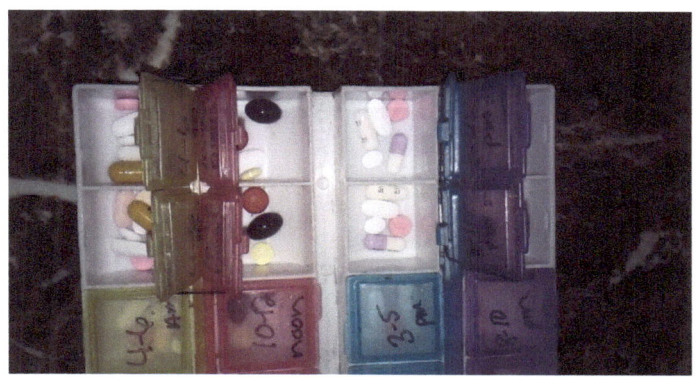

Medication changes a lot.

Diabetes how it can control your life

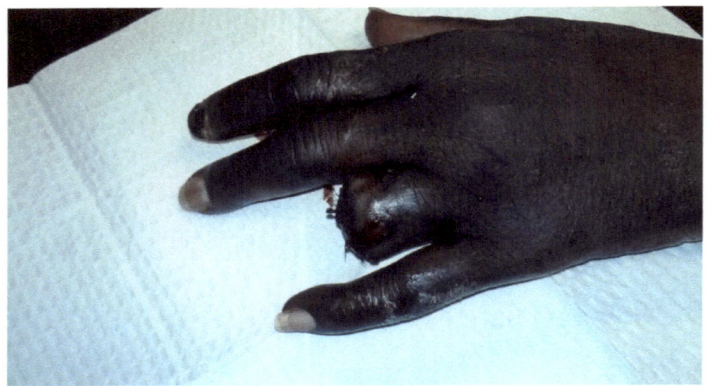

This is the finger they wanted to just rot off, another doctor took it off, but wow watch the results.

Tammy Thomas

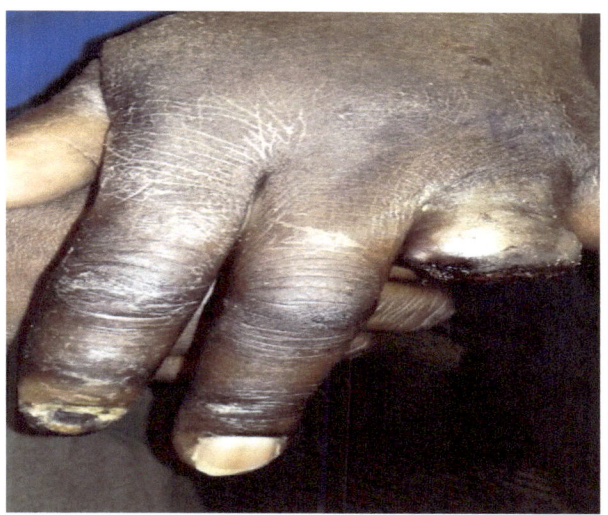

Once they start cutting it seems like it never end

Diabetes how it can control your life

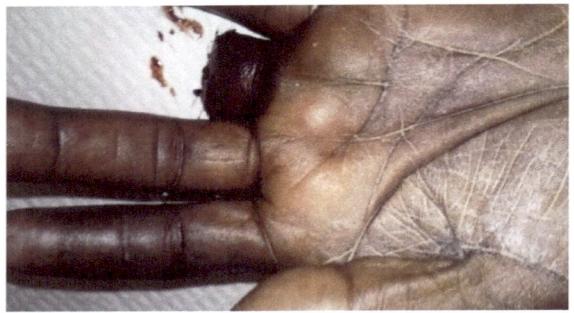

Tammy Thomas

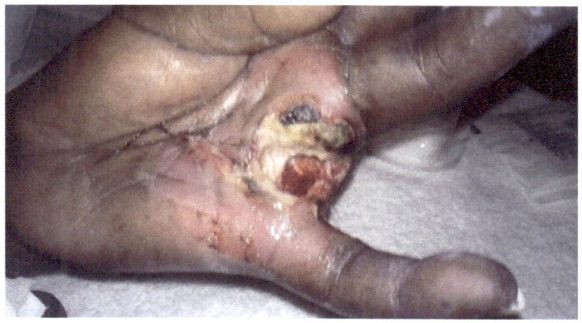

My current situation with finger 1

Diabetes how it can control your life

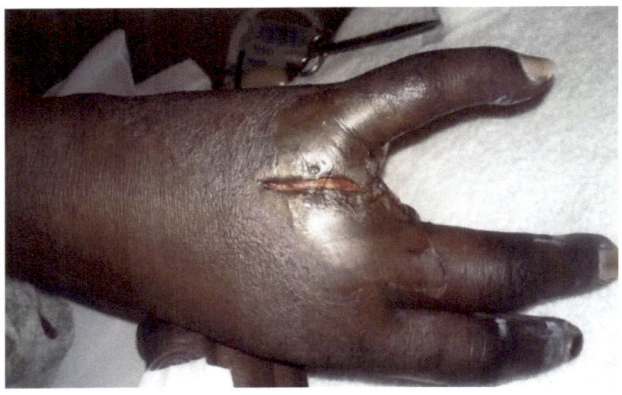

My current situation with my finger 2

Tammy Thomas

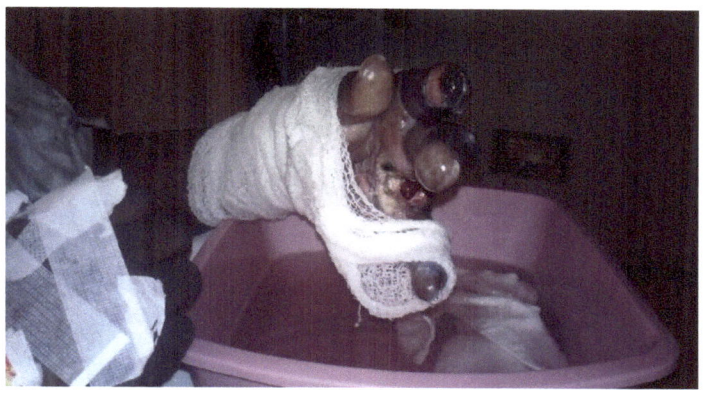

My current situation with my finger 3 Soaking it up to 3 times a day to try and save my mom hand.

Diabetes how it can control your life

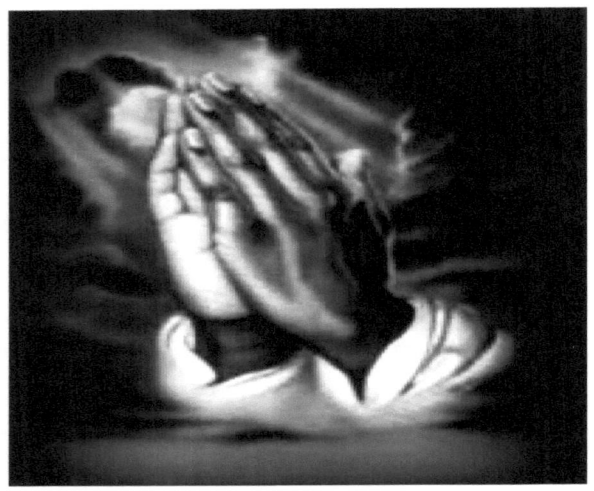

Pray

Tammy Thomas

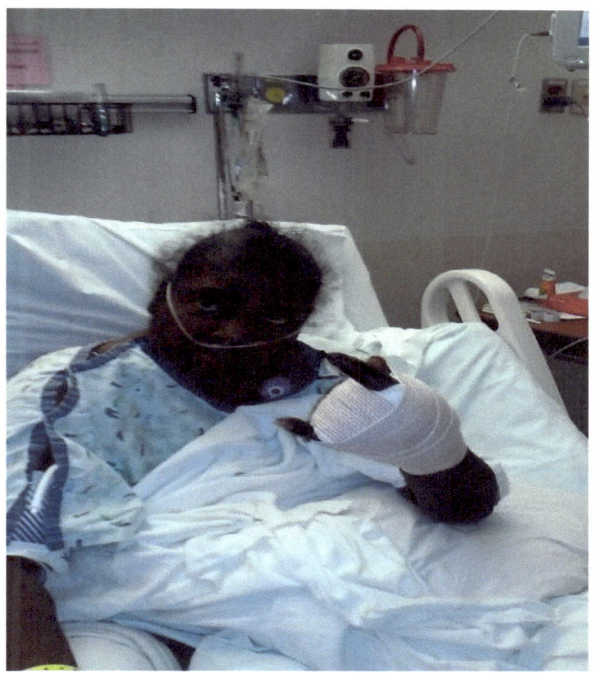

Last night they took off another finger

I could continue to go on and on but I'll stop here I hope that you take the time to get yourself under control much love S.F.L

Diabetes how it can control your life

Diabetes

I wish I know how strong you were

I would have never called your bluff

Now I see that my life is as clear as death can be.

So now all I do is huff and puff

I sit, I cry and ask god why

As I fall to my knees and look at the sky,

Oh lord please spare me,

For I love myself more than the can see.

I wish I know how strong you were,

I would have never called your bluff,

Now I see that my life is as clear as death can

So now all I do is huff and puff.

Tammy Thomas

I get tired,

I get stressed,

But in the end God knows best.

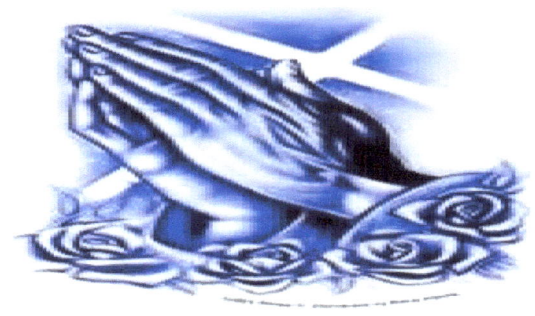

References

Healthy Living – mayoclinic.org American Diabetes Associate's – http://www.diabetes.org Diabetes, Digestion and Kidney Disease – http://www.niddk.nih.gov

Tammy Thomas

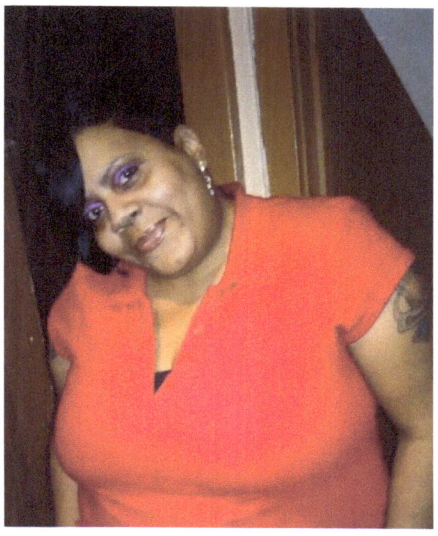

No matter what life throws at me I just pick up the pieces and keep it moving Thank you Jesus for keeping me strong and being able to deliver my messages through your guidance.

www.ingramcontent.com/pod-product-compliance
Lightning Source LLC
Chambersburg PA
CBHW040923180526
45159CB00002BA/593